Aboriginal Global Pioneers
Book 5

Australian Aboriginal Medicine

Caring for People

Marji Hill

Published by The Prison Tree Press 2024
Copyright © 2024 Marji Hill

The Prison Tree Press
Suite 124
1-10 Albert Avenue
Broadbeach, Queensland 4218
https://marjihill.com
https://www.fastselfpublishing.com

Disclaimer:
All the material contained in this book is provided for educational and informational purposes only. No responsibility can be taken for any results or outcomes resulting from the use of this material.

While every care has been taken to trace and acknowledge copyright the publishers tender their apologies for any accidental infringement where copyright has proved untraceable.

Every attempt has been made to provide information that is both accurate and effective, however, the author does not assume any responsibility for the accuracy or use/misuse of this information.

Acknowledgement is given to Canva for most of the illustrations in this book.

A catalogue record for this work is available from the National Library of Australia

Aboriginal Global Pioneers (Series of 5 Books)

ISBN 978-1-7637384-0-9 Hardback
ISBN 978-1-7637384-1-6 eBook

Australian Non-Fiction | First Nations | History

Acknowledgements

I acknowledge the Traditional Custodians of Country
throughout Australia
and their connections to land, sea, and community.

I pay my respect to elders, past, present, and emerging
and extend my respect to all First Nations peoples today.

In the spirit of reconciliation,
my mission is to increase understanding
between the First Nations and other Australians
and to provide people from all over the globe
some basic understanding of Australia's first people,
their history, and cultures.

Marji Hill

Contents

INTRODUCTION

In Western societies, medical practitioners (doctors) help to heal people who are ill. They diagnose the cause of the illness and then treat it.

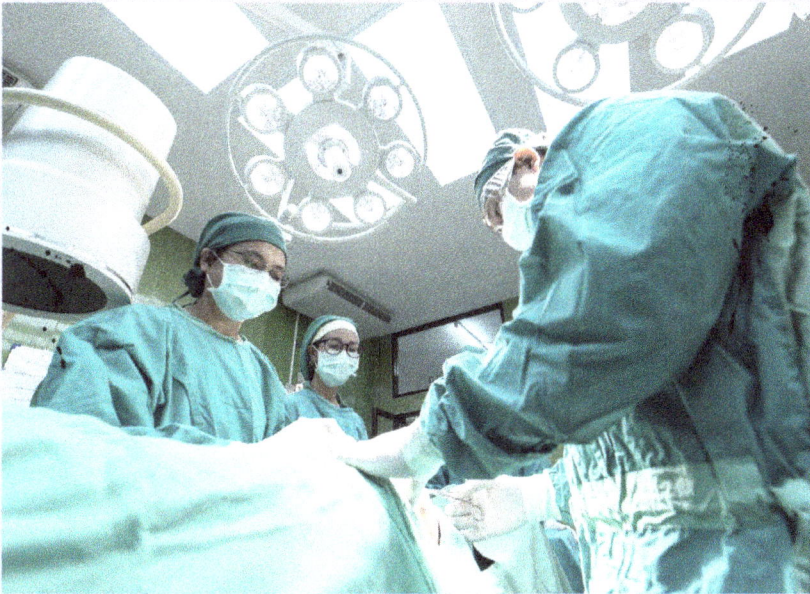

Medical practitioner

Australia's First Nations people also have doctors who diagnose and treat those who are ill.

They are called traditional healers.

They are global pioneers in medicine. Their healing practices are not just about treating physical ailments.

First Nations doctors understand the spiritual and emotional needs of their patients.

They draw on ancient religious and spiritual beliefs in combination with natural remedies which come from their intimate knowledge of natural substances like bush medicines.

These ancient healing practices have been passed down through generations, giving us a rich history of bush medicines and spiritual insights that continue to be relevant today.

First Nations traditional healers are also known by other names such as "clever men", "medicine men," or "men of high degree".

First Nations societies place great faith in their traditional healers. These people have special powers derived from their spiritual Ancestors to cure the sick.

Traditional healers can "see" into the body of their patients.

They deal with physical, spiritual and emotional problems and their role is similar to the general practitioner or a psychiatrist in the Western world.

Australia's First Nations people are made up of many cultures all of which have their own healing practices.

These vary and may include special rituals and ceremonies for healing, smoking ceremonies, massage, the application of ochre and clay, going to special healing sites, healing stones, physic or energy healing, meditation, and bush medicines.

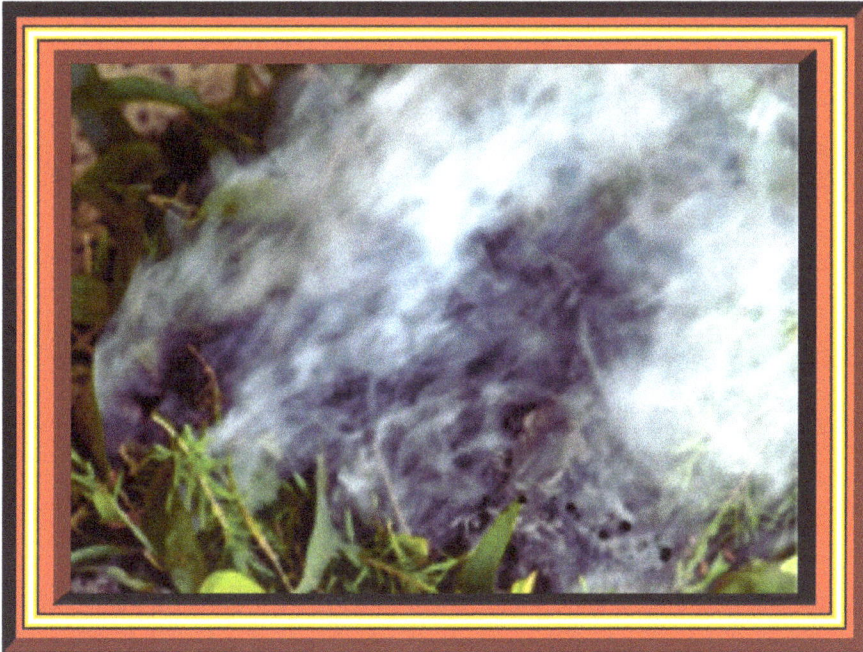

Smoking ceremony

TRADITIONAL HEALERS

First Nations traditional healers are very special people who are held in high regard by their people.

Usually they are men but there are healers who are women. These spiritual doctors possess great wisdom and have special stature and power.

Some women with outstanding intellect are admitted to the special knowledge of traditional healers.

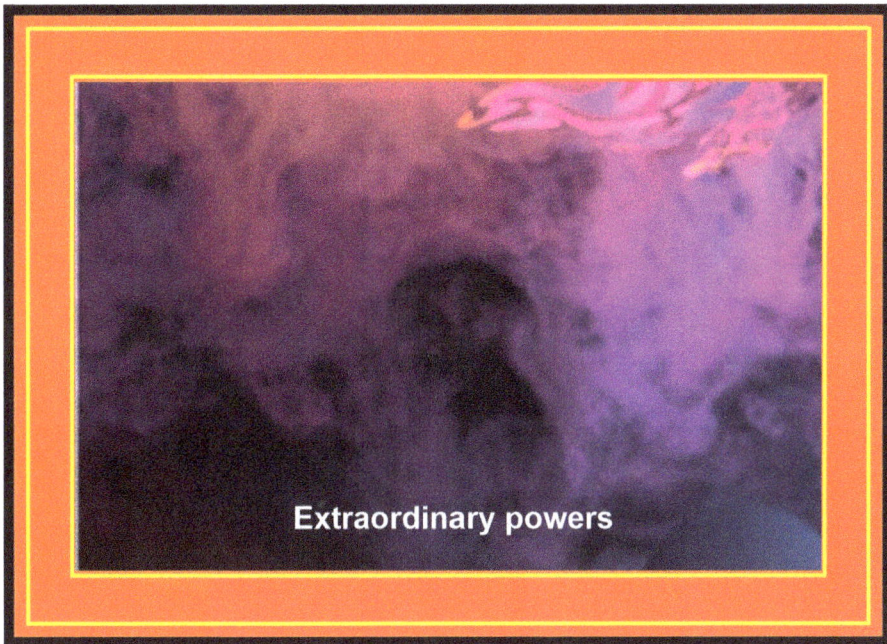

Extraordinary powers

While any First Nations person may prepare and use bush medicine, the traditional healers have exceptional knowledge and very special powers.

Their powers are extraordinary particularly in the realm of the supernatural: they can divine and interpret the symptoms of illness, cure, mysteriously kill, fly and travel over the land at great speed, anticipate events, practise telepathy, make rain, know what is happening in faraway places, communicate with Ancestral beings and see spirits and ghosts of the dead.

Their powers include divination, massage, and the extraction of "objects" that have been inserted into a victim by sorcery. Healing songs, special crystals and healing stones are all part of their medical kit.

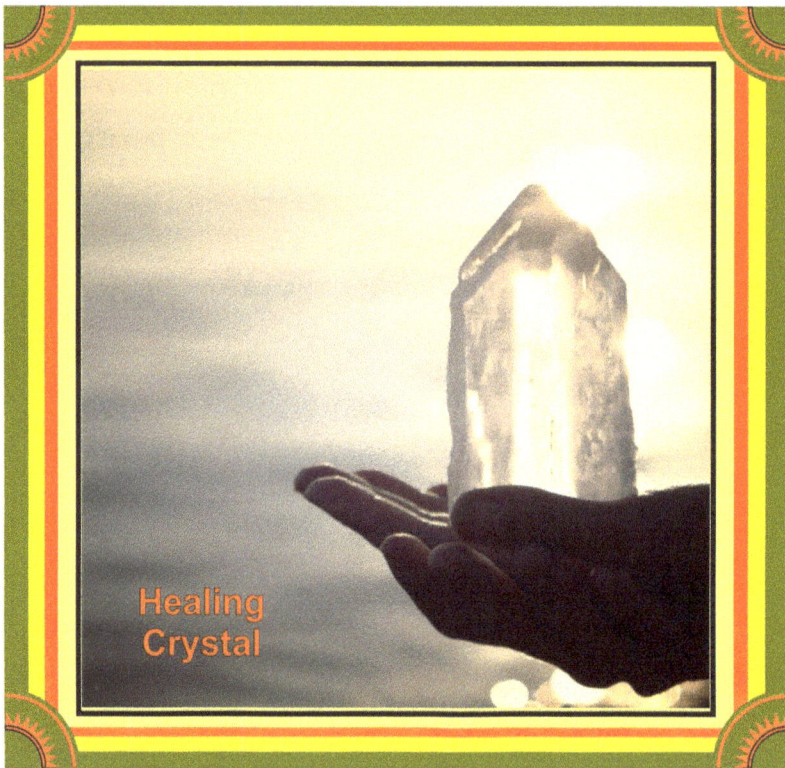

Healing Crystal

The traditional healer has a variety of healing treatments including bush rubs and bush medicines. They are intent on healing the physical body and the mind, and comforting and instilling faith into the ones in their care.

They give reassurance to the patient and provide explanations as to why someone is sick, just as happens in Western medicine.

Some traditional healers inherit their special powers, their knowledge being passed down from generation to generation. They may have been born into it, the process starting when a child is identified by both their family and community as having special healing qualities.

Other healers acquire their skills through being an apprentice. They are initiated into the secrets and become the supreme authorities on spiritual matters. This involves special training, commencing when a person is young and involves spiritual revelation.

When a person is sick, a traditional healer promotes an atmosphere around the sick person which helps them regain their faith and confidence. They help a person's psychological welfare by providing positive emotional support.

The role of the traditional healer has been likened firstly to that of a priest who instils faith, secondly a bit like a Western doctor who cures the sick and thirdly, like a coroner who tries to determine the cause of the illness or death.

CAUSES OF ILLNESS

The causes of illness and death in Western societies is largely due to natural causes. There are usually a number of factors that contribute to illness such as obesity, lack of exercise, smoking, excessive alcohol, and poor diet. A headache, for example, may be due to stress, high blood pressure, or a lack of water.

In First Nations cultures, however, the cause of illness and death lies largely in the realm of the supernatural.

Sorcery and the supernatural are part of the perceived reality of people in First Nations cultures.

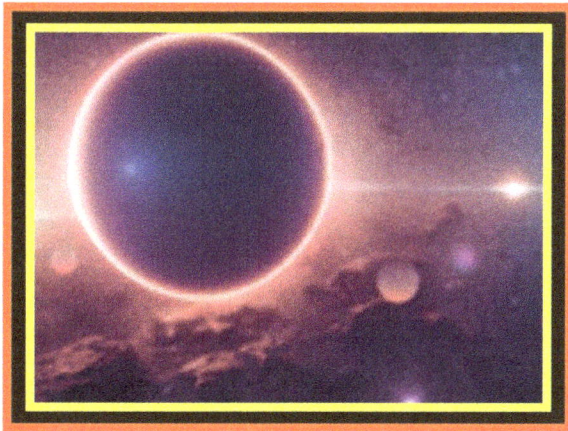

Supernatural intervention

Supernatural intervention plays a very important role in the traditional health beliefs as it may provide the "ultimate" reason why a person became ill.

A person could be ill because they have broken a taboo, entered a dangerous and sacred site thus upsetting the spirit forces or power emanating from that location. They may have angered an Ancestral spirit by being in a place where they should not be.

Having an accident, such as falling out of a tree or breaking a bone, may be caused by someone with evil intentions towards the injured person.

It is possible for the sick person to get better once the spiritual or supernatural cause of the illness has been removed.

However, the death of a baby or a very old or chronically ill person is regarded differently. Illness and death is explained in terms of natural causes. It's considered to be normal.

Certain ailments such as a headache, diarrhoea, infected eyes, and toothache are common and there are well established remedies. Some of these ailments are believed to be caused by seasonal changes.

Beliefs about health and illness are moulded by ancient cultural beliefs and traditions. A headache, for instance, could be caused by the coming of cold winds. All is well once a person's distress has disappeared.

But more serious illness or death may have a supernatural cause, especially if it is premature, unexpected or sudden.

SORCERY

Traditional healers are trained to remove the influence of sorcery and evil spirits and to restore the wellbeing of the soul or spirit.

Sorcery is when someone with evil intent causes harm to others through the performance of certain rites.

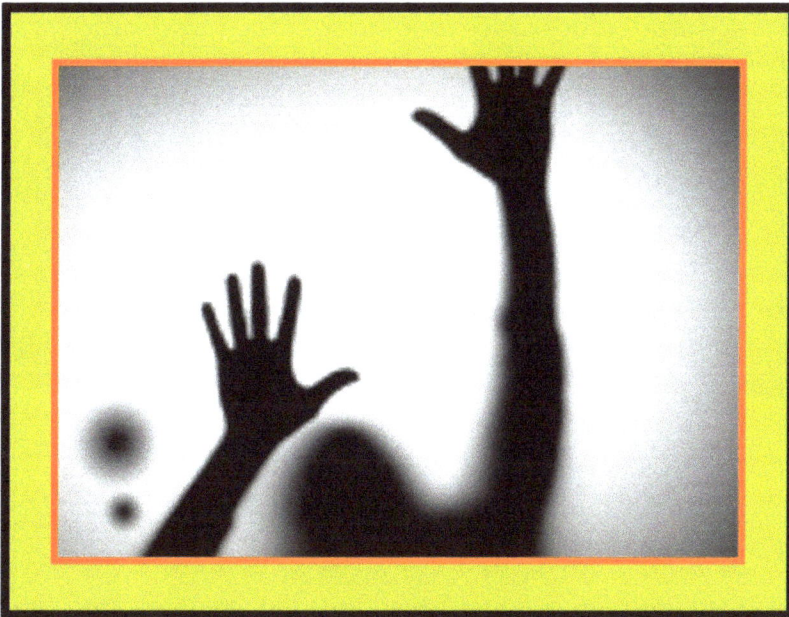

Sorcery

A victim could be waylaid in the bush, overpowered and rendered unconscious. A sharp object is believed to be inserted into the body. Once this is completed the victim returns to normal, goes back to the camp but within a few days falls ill and dies.

Sorcerers can cause illness and death by projecting an evil spirit or "object" into a person by "pointing the bone". This is a common practice. A victim of bone pointing sickens and dies unless a traditional healer is called in to remove the evil powers that are causing the illness.

There are many techniques of sorcery practice. Anything which has a close association with the person such as a piece of hair, nail clippings, body fluids, hair or food can be used by a sorcerer to harm or kill their victim.

In Central Australia, sorcerers wear *kurdaitja* shoes made of feathers and blood to conceal their footprints. Crystals, pebbles, quartz, pearl shells and many kinds of ornaments and charms are used to cause illness and death.

Sorcery is a cause of illness and death just as are breaches of religious sanctions and social rules of behaviour. A person may have broken cultural laws, lost their soul, or become victim of a psychic attack.

Sorcerers are universally feared in First Nations societies. It is still a potent belief and the casting and removal of evil spells is still practised today.

If illness is believed to be caused by sorcery the traditional healer is trained to remove the influence of sorcery and to restore the wellbeing of the soul or spirit.

Once the spiritual or supernatural cause of the illness has been withdrawn then it is possible for the sick person to get better.

Supernatural intervention plays a very important role in the traditional health beliefs of First Nations people as it may provide the 'ultimate' reason why a person became ill.

TRADITIONAL MEDICINE TODAY

Traditional medicine is still practised in many areas today. The extent to which it is practised varies widely amongst communities throughout Australia.

A health initiative is taking place in Anangu Pitjintjatjara Yangkunjatjara (APY) country in the northern part of South Australia.

Here there is a health care model designed to help traditional health care services to work hand-in-hand with western medicine.

Traditional health and medicine is alive and well in this region.

Anangu traditional healers of the Western Desert in Central Australia are called *Ngangkari*. Ngangkari are increasingly being brought into Western health settings to work with Western doctors.

If a Ngangkari is recognised as having particular powers for healing in childhood they are then encouraged to develop their skills. They often talk about being taught by their grandparents.

Ngangkari healing includes techniques such as observing, listening and touch.

They use massage and release "blockages" from the body and when required, they apply various herbal tinctures and ointments.

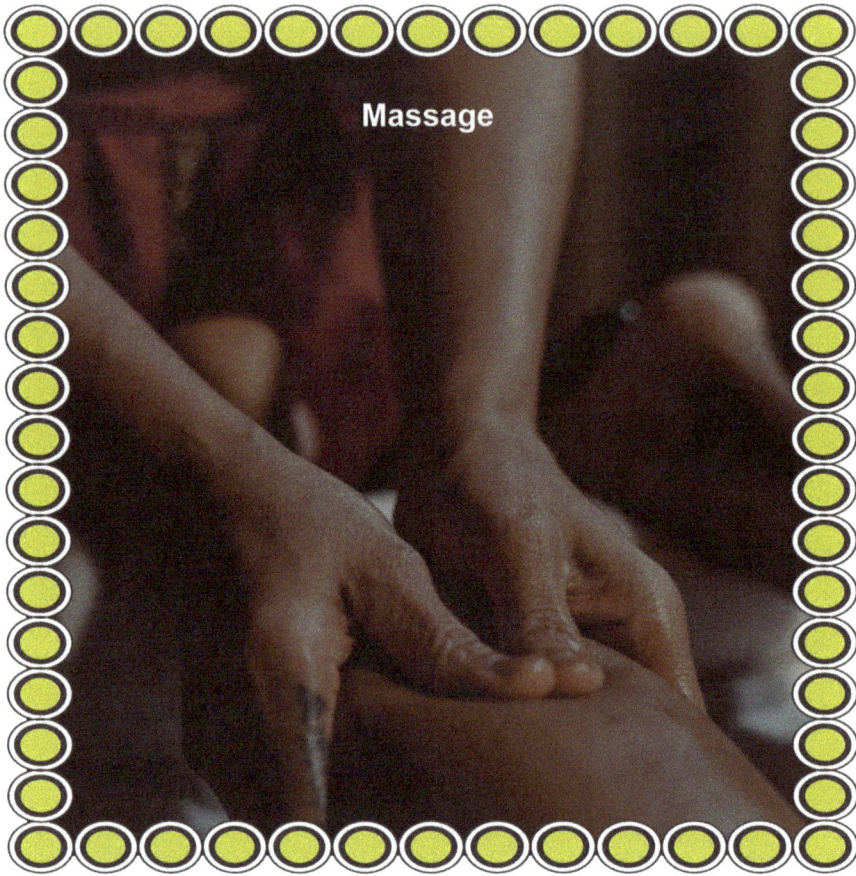

Massage

There is an understanding that the spirit can become dislodged through trauma, causing mental and physical disorders. Ngangkari bring it back into place. They are particularly adept at treating psychological disorders.

COMMON AILMENTS

Plants play an important role in all bush medicine practices.

Many plants have proven results in healing or for preventing disease. They are used to relieve symptoms of fever, congestion, headache, skin sores, aching limbs and digestive problems.

Plants found in Australian suburban gardens today are recognised for their medicinal benefits.

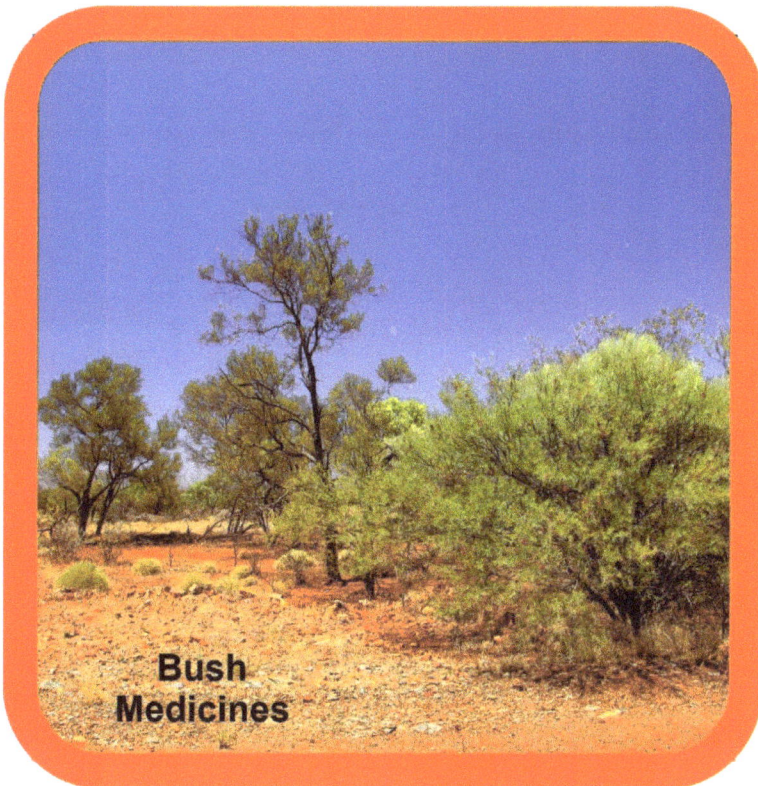

Bush Medicines

Bush medicines are part of the approach to healing and wellness in First Nations societies. For thousands of years, these natural remedies have been used to treat a variety of illnesses. Many remedies are still being used today.

Present day practitioners of bush medicine offer a wealth of knowledge that can be used to improve our understanding of the process of healing.

Just as in Western societies, people suffer ailments like a toothache, headache, aches and pains, bites and stings, burns, eye infections, stomach upsets, stings, snake bites, constipation or diarrhoea. These are all treatable with bush remedies.

Remedies vary throughout the continent. There is not one set of bush medicines or remedies.

Bush remedies can include drinks, washes, massages and aromatherapies.

The smell of some plants can be infused through steam and smoke. A drink potion can be made by heating water with plant additives.

Plants may be boiled and once the liquid is cooled it can be either imbibed or applied externally to the body.

Some plants are heated, rubbed or massaged into an affected part of a patient's body.

Bark from the leopard-wood tree was used to cure aching teeth, whitewood gum was used for diarrhoea, and pelican oil was applied to burns.

Many preparations from plants could be used to treat ailments such as colds, fever, dysentery, toothache, sore ears and so on. The bark of eucalyptus was soaked in water and swallowed to cure dysentery; melaleuca leaves were bruised in water and the resulting liquid was a cure for coughs, colds, and congestion.

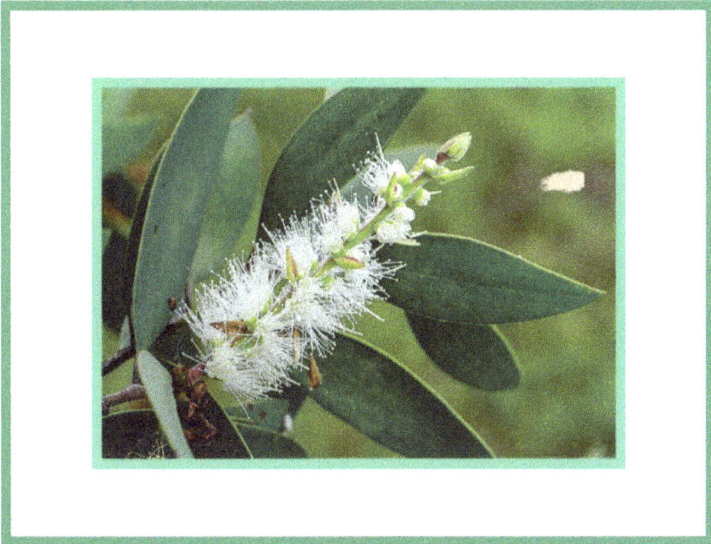

Many preparations from plants could be used to treat ailments

Various kinds of fat mixed with mud was used as a dressing for cuts and wounds. Eucalyptus was boiled into a pulp and applied to bruises, sprains, aches and pains.

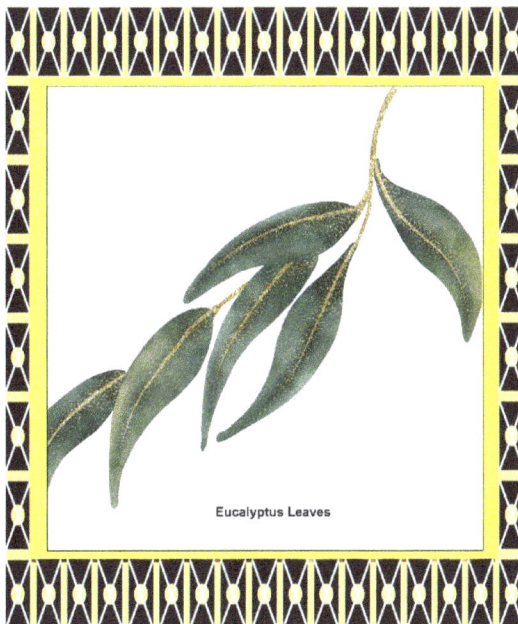

Eucalyptus Leaves

If, however, a person's illness is serious then a traditional healer will be called in to administer to the patient in a ritual manner.

As keen observers of the environment, First Nations people knew their botany and were aware of the medicinal properties of various species and plants.

Present day practitioners of bush medicine offer a wealth of knowledge that can be used to improve our understanding of the process of healing.

For common ailments in Western societies, a patient will go to the chemist and will purchase appropriate tablets, lotions, or some sort of remedy.

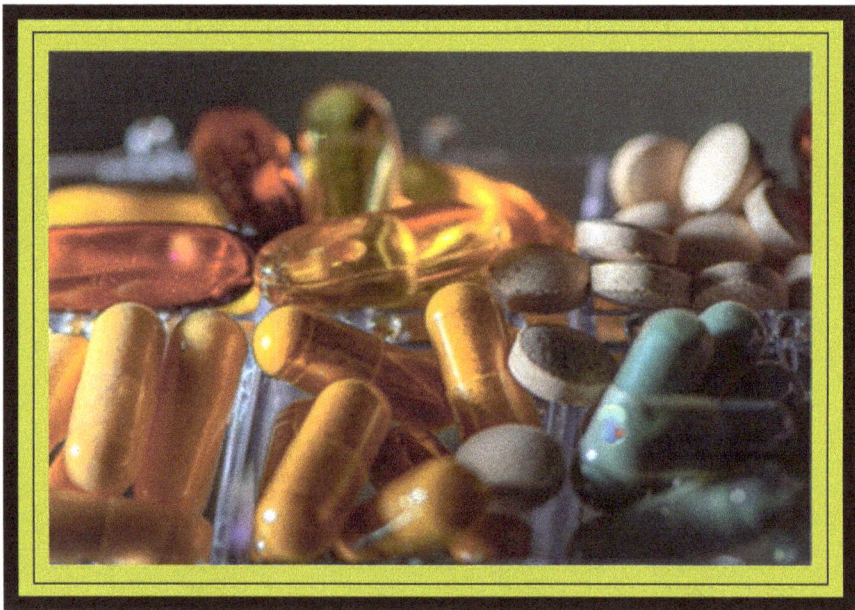

**In Western societies a patient will go to the chemist
to purchase appropriate tablets**

Likewise, most First Nations people have a basic knowledge of their bush remedies such as herbs, animal products, steam baths, charcoal and mud. As already discussed, healing in First

Nations societies involves not only just common bush medicines but also the spiritual.

SOME BUSH REMEDIES

Among Australia's First Nations cultures maintaining health was based upon cultural beliefs of the causes of sickness and the powers of their remedies. The causes of serious illness were generally attributed to supernatural sources. But just as in Western societies everyday remedies were derived from plants.

Healing among First Nations people involves the mind, body, and spirit. The approach to medicine is holistic in that it aims to restore balance in a person.

Here is a short list of some of the common bush remedies:

Vitamin C deficiency - Kakadu plum (*Terminalia ferdinandiana*) is recognised as the richest source of Vitamin C in the world. It is found in the bush of the Northern Territory and Western Australia.

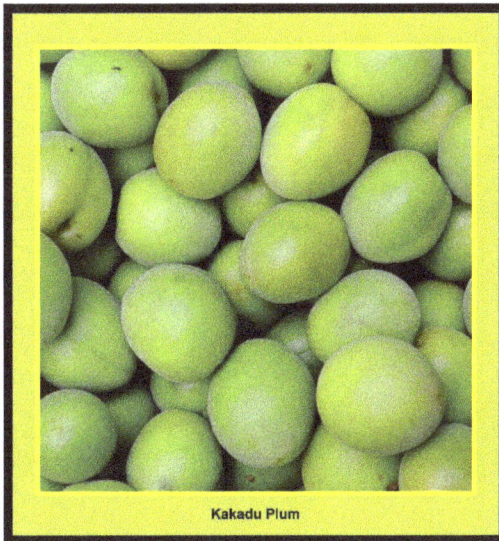

Kakadu Plum

Wounds - Bundjalung people from the coast of New South Wales crushed tea-tree (or paper bark) leaves and applied the paste to wounds as well as brewing it to a kind of tea for throat ailments.

Burns - Witchetty grubs are not only a good source of food but they can be crushed into a paste and placed on burns and covered with a bandage to seal and soothe the skin.

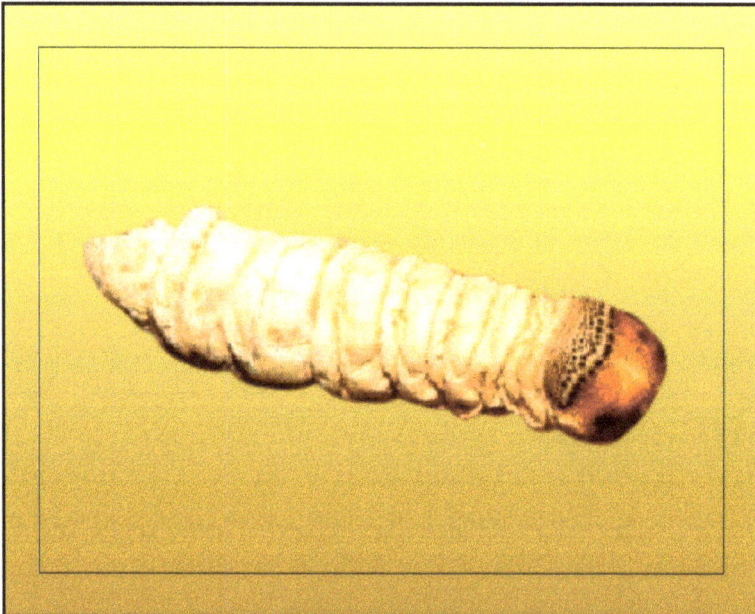

Witchetty grubs

Aching joints - Kangaroo apple (*Solanum aviculare* or *Solanum laciniatum*) is a natural anti-inflammatory steroid which aids the production of cortisone. It is beneficial for treating aching joints and wounds. It also encourages skin rejuvenation on scarring, pigmentation and aging. Its fruit contains high levels of the alkaloid solanine which can be infused from the leaves with hot water to create steroids.

Sleep - In Australia there are more than one thousand wattle species. Wattle blossom was hung in people's dwellings to promote sleep. In Victoria, the bark of blackwood (*Acacia melanoxylon*) was infused and used to bathe rheumatic joints or ingested as a mild sedative for rheumatism or indigestion.

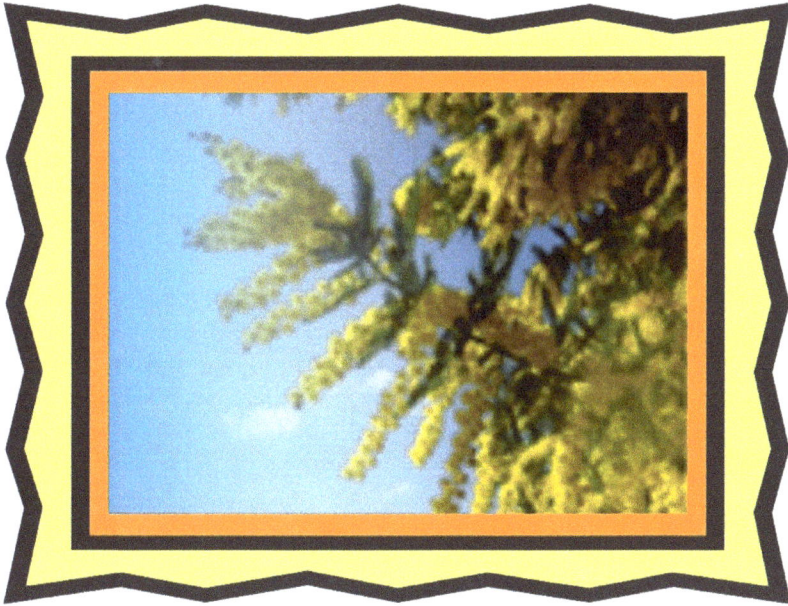

Wattle

Eye infections - Old man's weed (*Centipeda cunninghamii*) is used for treating things like eye infections, tuberculosis and skin complaints. It is commonly found along the Murray River as well as in other low-lying, swampy habitats,. It is administered as an extract in water, or sometimes rubbed onto the skin.

It's usually used for colds and coughs and chest infections, but, being a natural restorative plant, it can help strengthen the immune system and mobility.

Rheumatism - Drooping she-oak (*Allocasuarina verticillata*) has mature cones which when ground up can be applied to sores to treat rheumatism.

Toothache & cuts - Hop bush (*Dodonaea viscosa*) is a plant that grows across Australia. In Queensland the juice of the root is applied to toothache and cuts. The chewed leaf and juice were put on stonefish and stingray stings and bound up for four or five days.

Colds -Eucalyptus has antibacterial and analgesic properties, so is good for treating colds and respiratory problems, joint and muscle pain, dental health, fungal infections and wounds. Its scent is also a brilliant, natural insect repellent.

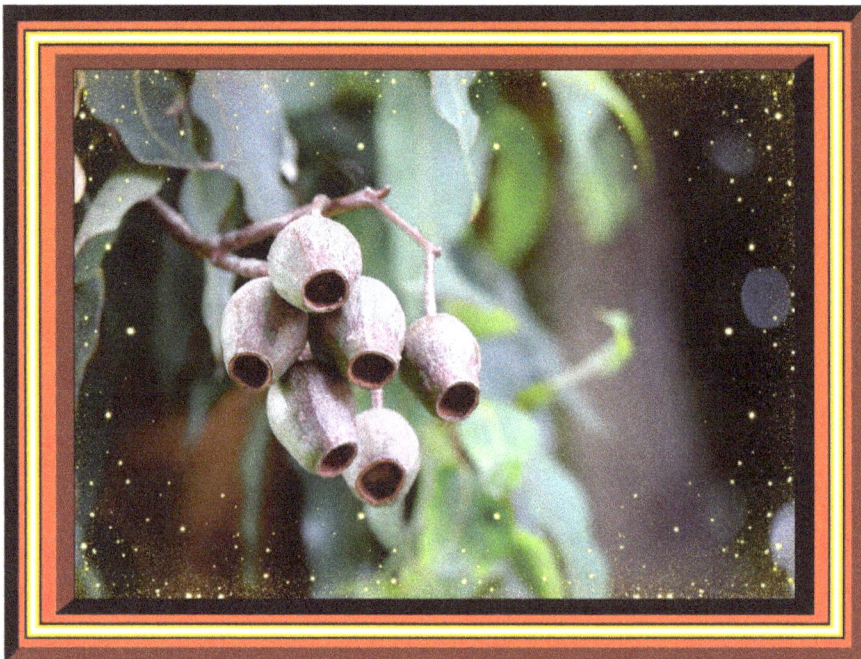

Eucalyptus gumnut

Glossary

Aromatherapy   Using sweet smelling substances to help cure a person

Divination   The skill or act of saying or discovering what will happen in the future

Dysentery   A disease of the bowel that causes the contents to be passed out of the body much more often and in a more liquid form than usual. It is caused by an infection that is spread by dirty water or food

Steroid   An artificial form of a natural chemical substance that is used for treating particular medical conditions

Telepathy   Knowing what is in someone else's mind, or the ability to communicate with someone mentally, without using words or other physical signals

Sources

The author acknowledges the following sources of information.

Australian InFo International 1989 *Australian Aboriginal Culture*. Canberra, Australian Government Publishing Service

Elkin, A.P. 1977 *Aboriginal Men of High Degree*. 2nd ed. St Lucia, Qld, University of Qld Press.

Gott, Beth 2018 "The art of healing: five medicinal plants used by Aboriginal Australians" https://theconversation.com/the-art-of-healing-five-medicinal-plants-used-by-aboriginal-australians-97249

Hill, Marji 1978 *A Response to Illness: A Study Of The Traditional Practitioner in Aboriginal Australia.* Master of Arts (Qualifying) thesis, Canberra, Australian National University.

Hill, Marji 2021 *First People Then and Now: Introducing Indigenous Australians.* 2nd ed. Broadbeach, The Prison Tree Press.

https://www.friendsofglenthorne.org.au/wp-content/uploads/Clarke-Vol-33-2008.pdf

Lee, Bilawarra 2013 *Healing from the Dilly Bag: Holistic Healing for your Body, Soul, and Spirit*

Maher, Patrick 1999 "A Review of 'Traditional' Aboriginal Health Beliefs" Aust. Journal Rural Health, 7, 229–236

Williams, Victoria Grieves 2018 "Traditional Aboriginal healers should work alongside doctors to help close the gap" https://theconversation.com/traditional-aboriginal-healers-should-work-alongside-doctors-to-help-close-the-gap-93660

Who is Marji Hill

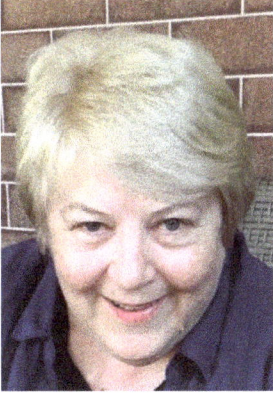

Marji Hill, artist and painter since childhood, runs her art career alongside her career as an author.

She is a highly respected international author as well as a seasoned business executive, researcher and coach.

Marji is passionate about promoting understanding between Australia's first people and other Australians.

The spirit of reconciliation was fostered in all her writings ever since she was a Research Fellow in Education at the Australian Institute of Aboriginal and Torres Strait Islander Studies (AIATSIS) in Canberra.

From 2008 to 2011, Marji was Deputy Chairperson of the Mosman Branch of Reconciliation Australia in Sydney.

Following her Research Fellowship at AIATSIS in 1976 Marji, together with her late partner, Alex Barlow, produced more than seventy (70) books on all aspects of the First Nations people including the critical, annotated bibliography *Black Australia*.

In 1989 she was the Project Coordinator and one of the researchers and writers of *Australian Aboriginal Culture* the official Australian Government publication on First Nations people.

In 1988 *Six Australian Battlefields* was published by Angus and Robertson. A decade later it was re-published by Allen & Unwin as a paperback edition.

Her nine-volume encyclopaedia, *Macmillan Encyclopaedia of Australia's Aboriginal Peoples* was published in 2000 and in 2009 she published *The Apology: Saying Sorry To The Stolen Generations.*

Marji's more recent publications extend to self-improvement and self-help with books like *Staying Young Growing Old* and *Inspired by Country* a self-help book about painting with gouache.

More Books by Marji Hill

First Nations

Hill, Marji 2021 *Australian Aboriginal History: 5 Stories of Indigenous Heroes.* Broadbeach, Qld, The Prison Tree Press.

Hill, Marji 2021 *First People Then and Now: Introducing Indigenous Australians.* 2nd ed. Broadbeach, Qld, The Prison Tree Press.

Aboriginal Global Pioneers

Hill, Marji 2024 *Australian Aboriginal Origins: Earliest Beginnings.* Broadbeach, Qld, The Prison Tree Press. (Book 1)

Hill, Marji 2024 *Australian Aboriginal Trade: Sharing Goods and Services.* Broadbeach, Qld, The Prison Tree Press. (Book 2)

Hill, Marji 2024 *Australian Aboriginal Religion: Country and Dreaming.* Broadbeach, Qld, The Prison Tree Press. (Book 3)

Hill, Marji 2024 *Australian Aboriginal Fire: Managing Country.* Broadbeach, Qld, The Prison Tree Press. (Book 4)

Hill, Marji 2024 *Australian Aboriginal Medicine: Caring for People.* Broadbeach, Qld, The Prison Tree Press. (Book 5)

Self-improvement/Self-Help

Hill, Marji 2014 *Staying Young Growing Old.* Broadbeach, Qld, The Prison Tree Press.

Hill, Marji 2020 *How Big Is Your Why? An Author's Guide to Time Management and Productivity to Achieve Transformational Results.* Broadbeach, Qld, The Prison Tree Press.

Hill, Marji 2020 *A Create and Publish Toolbox: 101 Prompts In A Guided Journal To Help You Write, Self-publish, And Market Your Book On Amazon.* Broadbeach, Qld, The Prison Tree Press.

Hill, Marji 2021 *Inspired by Country: An Artist's Journey Back to Nature, Landscape Painting with Gouache.* Broadbeach, Qld, The Prison Tree Press.

Hill, Marji 2024 *Australian Paintings: Artworks by Marji Hill.* Broadbeach, Qld, The Prison Tree Press.

Gold

Hill, Marji 2022 *Gates of Gold: The Discovery of Gold, its Legacy and its Contribution to Australian Identity* Broadbeach, Qld, The Prison Tree Press.

Hill, Marji 2022 *Shadows of Gold: Eureka and the Birth of Australian Democracy.* Broadbeach, Qld, The Prison Tree Press.

Hill, Marji 2022 *Gold and the Chinese: Racism, Riots and Protest on the Australian Goldfields.* Broadbeach, Qld, The Prison Tree Press.

Hill, Marji 2022 *Ghosts of Gold: The Life and Times of Jupiter Mosman.* Broadbeach, Qld, The Prison Tree Press.

Hill, Marji 2022 *Blood Gold: Native Police, Bushrangers & Law and Order on the Goldfields.* Broadbeach, Qld, The Prison Tree Press.

www.ingramcontent.com/pod-product-compliance
Lightning Source LLC
Chambersburg PA
CBHW041602260326
41914CB00011B/1357